PHYSEO

TABLE OF CONTENTS

We would like to extend a special thanks to the following individual who have spent many hours tutoring, guiding and consulting this work, making Physeo Biostatistics possible.

Julie A. Hansen
Class of 2022
St. George's University SOM

BIOSTATISTICS

Section I - Biostatistics Overview

I. The whole purpose of biostatistics is to study disease and apply it to the patient.

A. Step 1: Design and perform a study.

1. Discussed in Section II.

B. Step 2: Evaluate the study.

1. Discussed in Sections II through V.

C. Step 3: Apply it to the patient.

1. Discussed in Sections VI through IX.

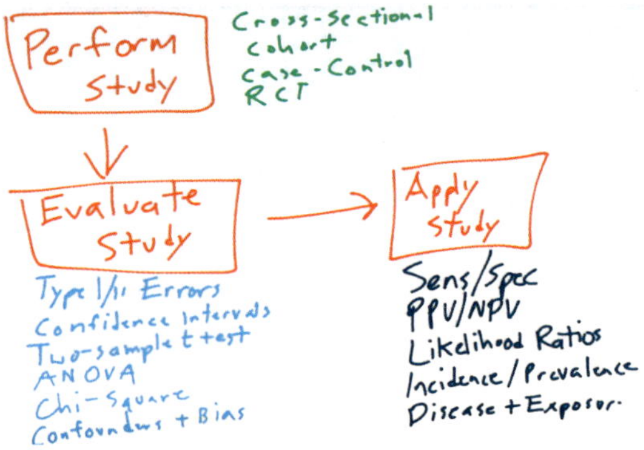

II. Mean: The average.

III. Median: The middle number.

IV. Mode: The most common number.

A. Very resistant to outliers.

B. Always the peak of the graph.

V. Normal Distribution

A. Mean = median = mode

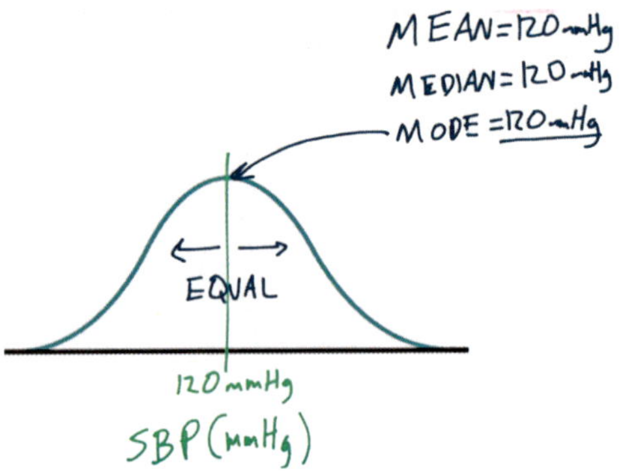

VI. Negative Skew

A. An abnormal distribution of data in which more data falls heavily on the left side, or more negative side of the graph.

Negative Skew

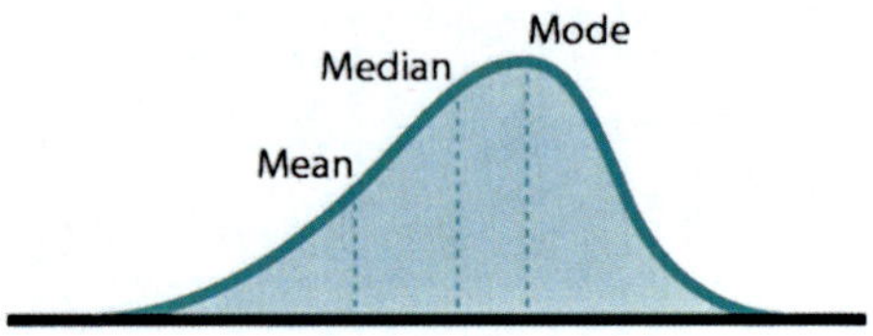

B. Organizing mean, median and mode

1. At the mode (peak), draw a line down the center of the graph. Notice more data falls on the left (negative) side.

2. Remember, "Mean, median, and mode" in that order.

a) Negative skew = more data on left = "mean, median, and mode" from left to right.

"Mean, Median, and Mode"

Negative Skew

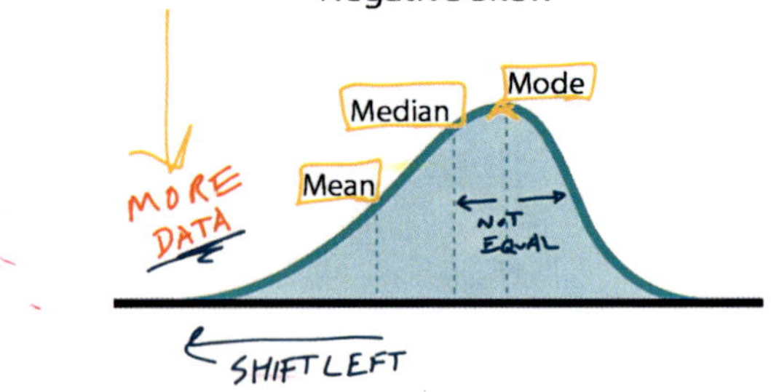

VII. Positive Skews

A. An abnormal distribution of data in which more data falls heavily on the right side, or more positive side of the graph.

Positive Skew

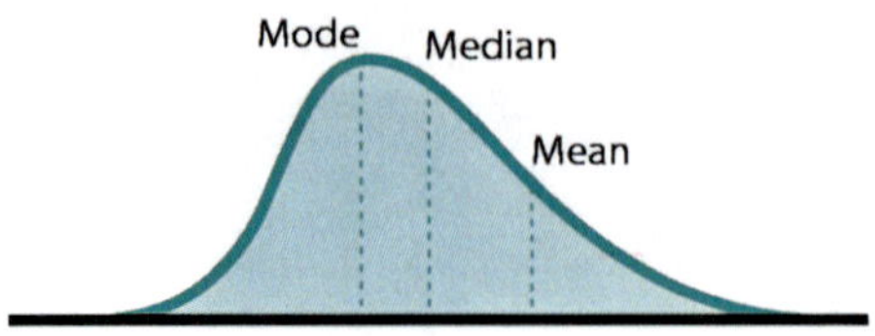

B. Organizing mean, median and mode

1. At the mode (peak), draw a line down the center of the graph. Notice more data falls on the right (positive) side.
2. Remember, "Mean, median, and mode" in that order.
   a) Positive skew = more data on right = "mean, median, and mode" from right to left.

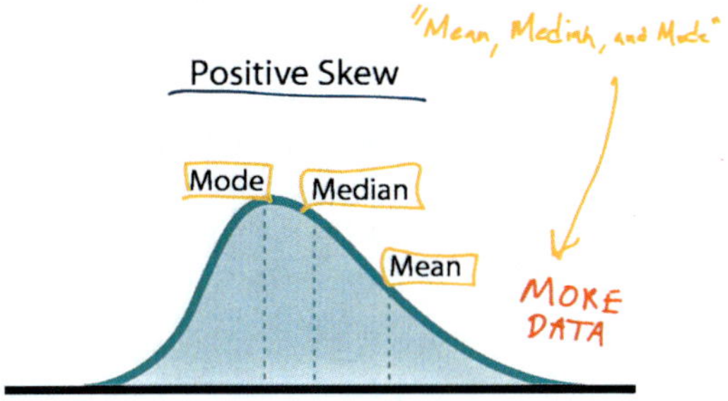

VIII. Standard Deviations (SD)

A. Represented by σ (sigma)

B. Measures the variability compared to the mean within a study set.

1. Higher SD indicates higher variability and higher dispersion (more results are distant from the mean).

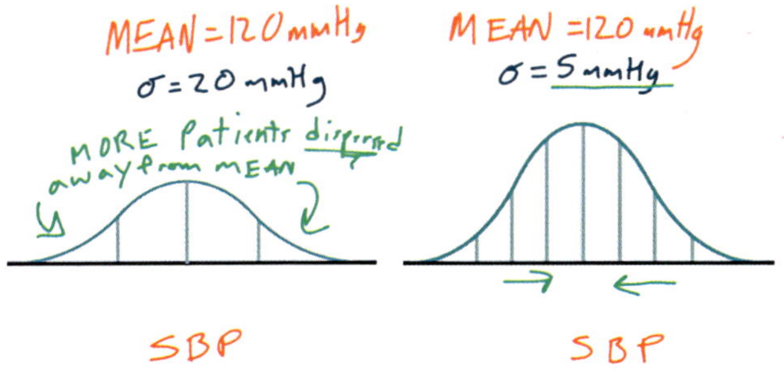

2. 1 SD = 68%
   a) Note: 32% of observations fall outside 1 SD (16% below and 16% above).
3. 2 SD (technically 1.96) = 95%
   a) Note: 5% of observations fall outside 2 SD (2.5% below and 2.5% above).
4. 3 SD (technically 2.58) = 99%
   a) Note: 1% of observations fall outside 3 SD (0.5% below and 0.5% above).

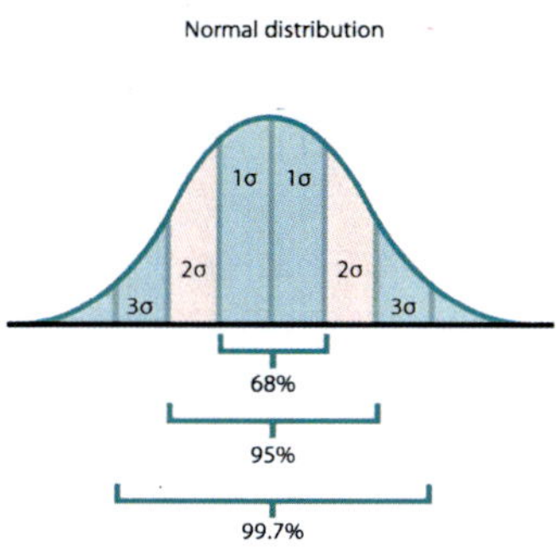

IX. Standard Error of the Mean (SEM)

A. Measures the variability between mean of sample and mean of general population.

B. σ / √*n*

1. ↑ n → ↓ SEM → ↓ variability (results cluster closer to the mean)
2. ↓ n → ↑ SEM → ↑ variability (results more dispersed)

X. Z-score

A. How many SD from the mean.

B. Example: 2 SD = Z score of 2.

REVIEW QUESTIONS

1. A study is performed in a family medicine clinic in which HbA1c is measured in otherwise healthy males between the ages of 20 and 30. The HbA1c results range from 4% to 5.3%. However, an unusual number of new patients have a HbA1c of 3% to 3.5%. How would the mean shift in relation to the median and mode?

   - **The new group is lower than that found on the original, normal distribution of patients → negative skew of data**
   - **Negative skew indicates more data on left → repeat, "mean, median, and mode" from left to right.**

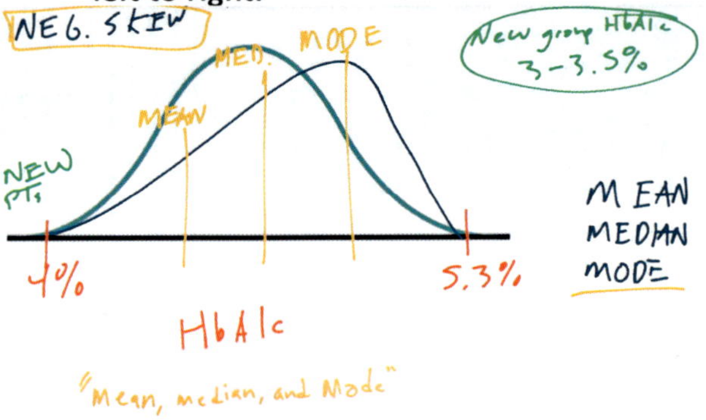

2. A study of 200 elderly males between the ages of 80-89 evaluates their cognitive ability with the MMSE. The average score out of 30 possible points is 23. One standard deviation is 2 points. How many patients have scores of 19 or lower?

   - **First, recognize that 19 is 2 standard deviations (SD) from the mean → 2 SD encompasses 95% of the data → 2.5% fall below this range → 0.025 x 200 patients = 5 patients**

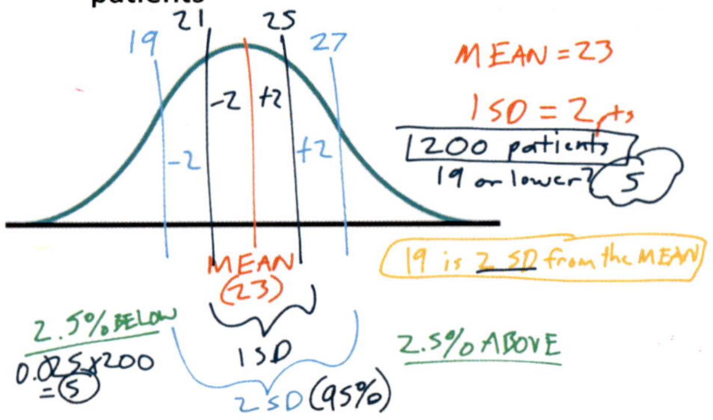

Section II - Study Designs

I. There are 7 study designs to be familiar with for board examinations.

Study Designs				
Study Type	**Starting Point**	**Mechanism**	**Finds**	**Prospective, Retrospective or Both?**
Cross-sectional	One population at a single point in time	Uses a single "snapshot" in time to study a population	- Disease prevalence - Correlation	Neither—it is performed at ONE single point in time
Cohort	2 cohorts (groups): 1) Experimental = group has risk factor or exposure 2) Control = group does NOT have risk factor or exposure	Follows 2 cohorts over time	- Incidence of disease (do more or less people w/ the risk factor or exposure develop disease?) - Relative risk (RR): likelihood of becoming diseased if you have a given risk factor or exposure	Both
Case-Control	2 groups: 1) Cases (experimental) = group has disease 2) Control = group does NOT have disease and matches in every other way to case group	Looks back in time to determine if cases were subjected to a given risk factor (or not)	- Odds ratio (OR): likelihood of having been exposed to a risk factor in the past if you have the disease	Retrospective
Randomized-Controlled Trial (RCT)	2 groups: 1) Treatment (experimental) = given drug or treatment of study 2) Placebo (control) = NOT given drug or treatment of study but instead a benign placebo	Observes whether a treatment is effective over time	- Causation	Prospective

Study Designs, continued				
Study Type	**Starting Point**	**Mechanism**	**Finds**	**Prospective, Retrospective or Both?**
Crossover Study	2 groups	RCT variant—each group receives treatment A or B for time X. After time X, each group switches treatment and uses it for time X. A washout period is used at the time patients switch treatments.	- Causation	Prospective
Case Series	1 group: diseased or treatment	Follows this group over time and documents disease progress or response to tx	- Disease or tx progress	Prospective
Ecological	Populations—usually w/a rare disease	Studies group factors (language, climate, etc) w/in a population	- Incidence - Prevalence - Correlation	Neither—at one point in time

II. Cross-Sectional Studies

A. A snapshot that determines disease prevalence (not incidence).

B. Can find correlation (not causation).

C. Does not follow participants over time.

Cross-Sectional Study

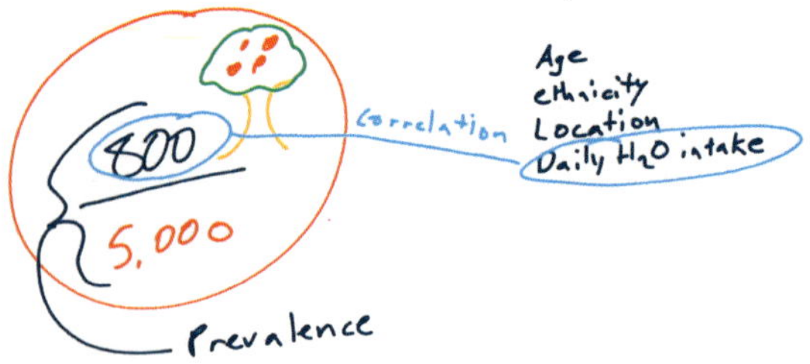

III. Cohort Study

A. 2 cohorts (groups) are followed over time.

B. Starting point = Exposure (risk factor).

C. Find a non-exposed control group.

D. Follow both groups over time and measure incidence of disease → determines relative risk (RR).

E. "You were exposed? Here is your relative risk of getting the disease."

F. Retrospective or prospective.

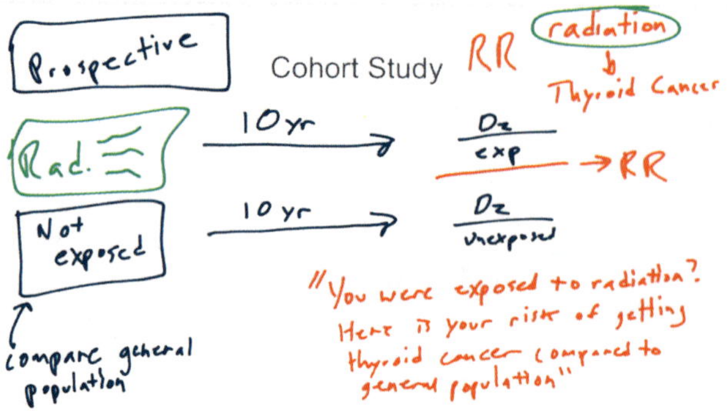

Case-Control Study

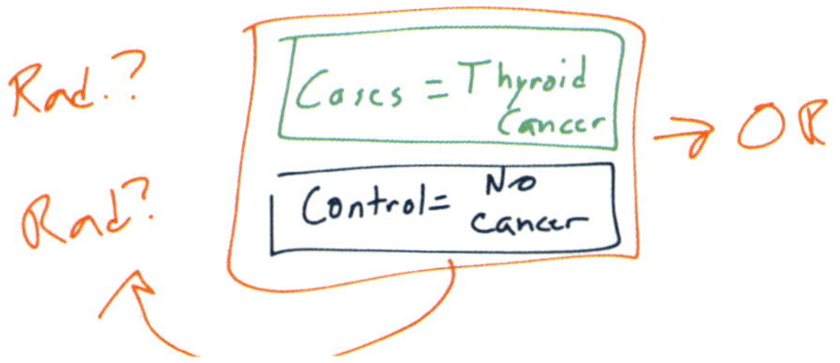

IV. Case-Control Study

A. 2 groups: Cases and controls

B. Starting point = Identify cases (diseased).

C. Find a non-diseased control group (prevents confounding).

1. The control should be the non-diseased, general population that matches in every other way to the case group.

2. Determine who was exposed in both groups → determines odds ratio (OR)

a) "You have the disease? Here are the odds you were exposed."

Case-Control Study

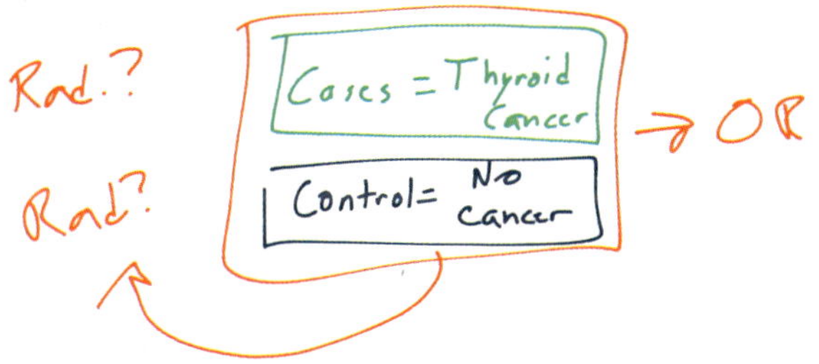

Case-Control versus Cohort

D. Cohort

1. Finds relative risk (RR)

2. Finds incidence

3. Starting point: Exposure → Follow to find disease

E. Case-Control

1. Finds odds ratio (OR)

2. Starting point: Disease (cases) → Go observe exposure

V. Randomized Controlled Trials (RCT)

A. Studies disease treatment.

B. Subjects randomly assorted to treatment or placebo group.

C. May involve single-blinding (subjects unaware of group status).

D. May involve double-blinding (subjects and physicians unaware).

E. Can identify causation but time-consuming and expensive.

Randomized-Controlled Trial (RCT)

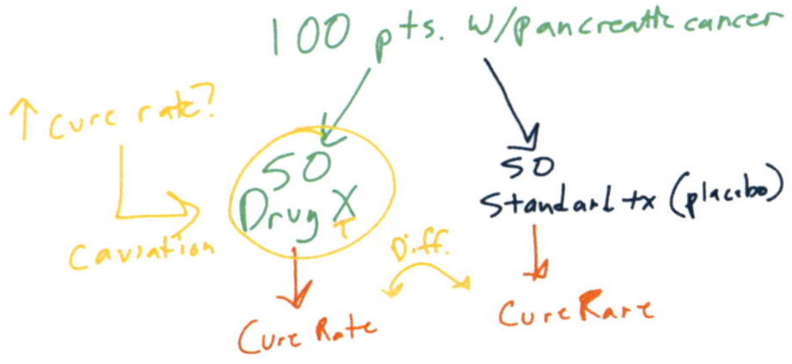

VI. Crossover Study

A. Variation of RCT → can determine causation.

B. Patients are randomly assorted to two groups.

C. Each receives treatment A or B for time X.

D. After time X, each group switches treatment and uses it for time X.

E. A washout period is often used at the time the patients switch treatments.

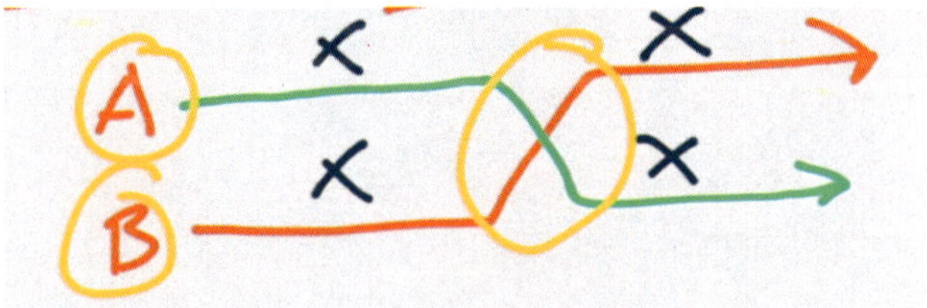

VII. Case Series

A. Identify diseased group → follows patients and documents their response to treatment or the progress of the disease.

VIII. Ecological Studies

A. Measures correlations among populations (not individuals).

B. Useful for very rare diseases.

C. Studies group factors (must be applied to the group).

1. Examples include climate, location, language, etc.

D. May identify incidence and prevalence at the population level.

E. Be careful not to apply results to individual patients (ecological fallacy).

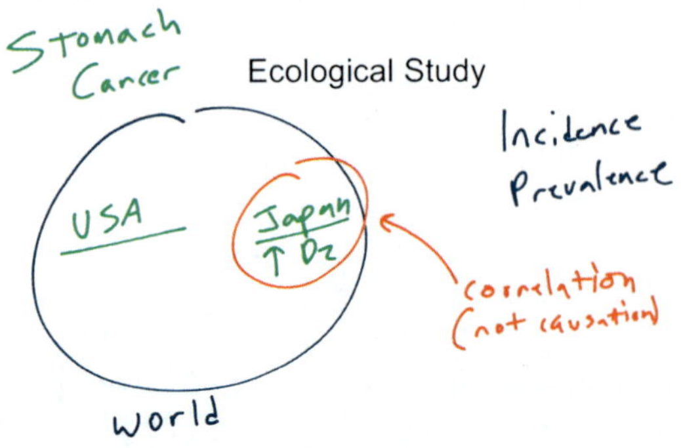

IX. Quick Guide

A. Cross-Sectional: Prevalence and correlation

B. Cohort: Incidence and RR

C. Case-Control: OR

D. Randomized Controlled Trial (RCT): Causation

E. Crossover Study: Causation

F. Case Series: Disease/treatment progress

G. Ecological Studies: Incidence, prevalence, and correlation

REVIEW QUESTIONS ?

1. A group of 125 people developed giardiasis in a city. The city officials suspected a contaminated water supply at the local reservoir as the cause. They surveyed everyone in the city to identify who had visited the reservoir over the past month. Officials were hoping to identify the incidence of giardiasis in their community over the past month. Would this be possible with this study model?

   - **First, recognize that this started with the group of cases and then went back to evaluate exposures in cases and controls (case-control study) → incidence cannot be found**
   - **Cohort studies start with exposed and non-exposed groups and identifies disease incidence in each group**

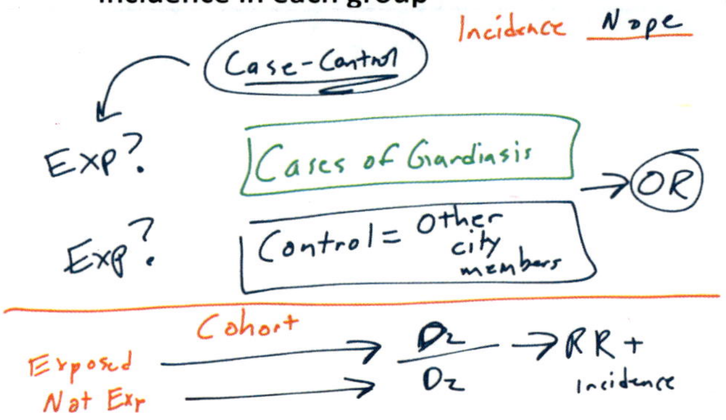

2. A single serum lead level was obtained in 1,000 participants in city A and 1,000 in city B. A positive level was considered above 5 micrograms/dL. Twelve participants in city A were positive and 400 participants were positive in city B. What type of study is this?

   - **A single lead level indicates a cross-sectional study → found correlation and prevalence**

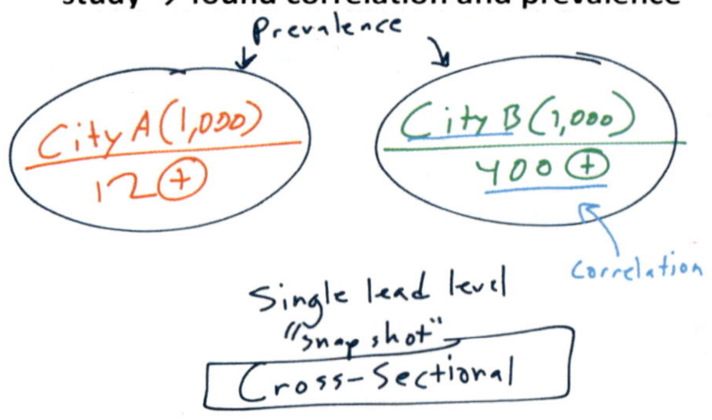

Section III - Evaluating Study Quality

I. Hypothesis Testing

A. Calculates the chance there is a true difference between two means.

1. i.e. The probability the difference observed was not due to chance.

B. H_0 = Null hypothesis (default: there is no association or difference)

C. H_1 = Alternative hypothesis (the one you are presenting: there is some association or difference)

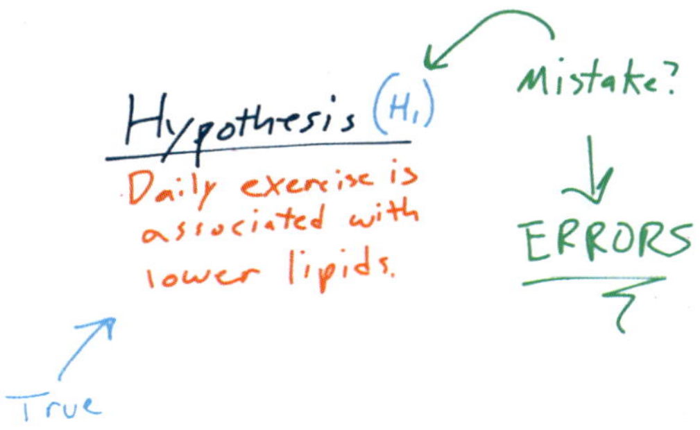

II. Type I (α) Errors

A. Incorrectly concluding that there is a difference (i.e. accepting alternative value H_1).

B. Probability of making type I error = α

C. α = *p* value

1. *p* value tells statistical significance.
2. Typically $p < 0.05$ (5%) which corresponds to 2 SD.

III. Type II (β) Errors

A. Incorrectly concluding that there is no difference (i.e. accepting H_0).

B. Increasing sample size (n) → decrease β error → increased power.

C. Power is the ability to detect a difference when there is one.

D. Power = 1 - β

IV. Type I (α) Errors versus Type II (β) Errors

A. When you accept H_0, think about β error and power.

B. When you accept H_1, think about α error and *p* value.

C. Mnemonic: "Bet0 power and alpha *p*"

V. Confidence intervals (CI)

A. How confident you are that the mean will fall within a given range.

B. CI = mean +/- z-score x (SEM)

C. Step 1: Identify the range

1. Range = mean +/- 1.96 x (SEM)
2. Example: 3.1 mg/dL +/- 1.2 mg/dL = Range (1.9 - 4.3 mg/dL)

D. Step 2: Identify the % that will fall within that range (usually 95%)

1. A 95% CI (2 SD) indicates p value of 0.05 (5%)
2. A 99% CI (3 SD) indicates p value of 0.01 (1%)

E. Example: 95% CI = 65 mg/dL +/- 0.87

F. Reject H_1 if CI range includes 1 (OR or RR)

1. Example: RR = 2 +/- 3 → -1 to 5 (includes 1)

G. Reject H_1 if CI range includes 0 (difference between means)

1. Example: 65 mg/dL - 58 mg/dL = 7 +/- 8 → -1 to 15 (includes 0)

REVIEW QUESTIONS

1. A group of non-dieting individuals is studied. The study concludes that daily aerobic exercise is associated with weight loss with a 7% chance they reached the conclusion incorrectly. Which hypothesis was rejected, the alternative or the null? Can you find the α or *p* value?

- **The question stem indicates that the alternative hypothesis (H_1) was accepted**
- **0.07 is the α**
- **0.07 is the *p* value**

H_1: Daily exercise (even if not dieting) is associated with weight loss ← Accepted (7% chance this was reached incorrectly)

H_0: The proposed hypothesis is wrong (there is no association)

α : 0.07

p : 0.07 (>0.05 is unacceptable)

2. A research group hypothesized that individuals that look at a computer screen within an hour of going to bed have a harder time falling asleep. After reviewing the data at the end of the study, the group determined there was no connection between computer screens and difficulty falling asleep. The power of the study was determined to be 0.96. Which hypothesis value did they accept? What is the chance they made a beta error?

- **Recall mnemonic: "Bet0 power and alpha *p*"**
- **The null hypothesis (H0) was accepted → think about β error and power**
- **Power = 1 - β → 0.96 = 1 - β**
- **β = 0.04 (4%)**

H_1 = Computer screen associated with difficulty falling asleep ← Rejected

H_0 = No connection ← Accepted

"Bet0 power and alpha *p*"

β = 0.04 (4%)
Power = 0.96 (96%)

3. A study is evaluating the LDL levels in 320 FBI applicants. Results show an average LDL level of 65 mg/dL with a standard deviation of 8 mg/dL. What would be the 95% confidence interval for this study?

- **95% CI = mean +/- z-score x SEM**
- **65 mg/dL +/- 1.96 x (8 mg/dL / √320)**
- **65 mg/dL +/- 087 (64.13 mg/dL to 65.87 mg/dL)**

65 mg/dL   95% = 2 SD 1.96 $\frac{\sigma}{\sqrt{n}} = \frac{8}{\sqrt{320}}$

95% CI = Mean +/- z-score x SEM

65 mg/dL +/- 1.96 x $\frac{8 \text{ mg/dL}}{\sqrt{320}}$

= 65 mg/dL +/- 0.87

95% CI = 64.13 mg/dL to 65.87 mg/dL

Section IV - Evaluation Study Significance

I. Statistical Tests

A. Useful to determine statistical significance ($p < 0.05$)

II. Two-sample t Test

A. Compares the means of 2 groups.

B. Used for numerical data.

Two-sample t test

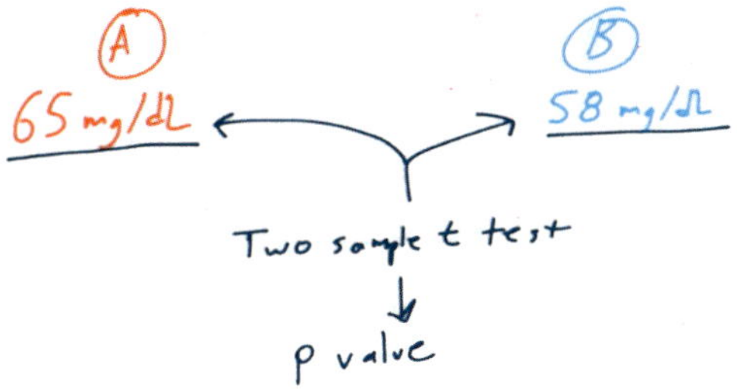

III. Analysis of Variance (ANOVA)

A. Compares the means of 2+ groups.

B. Used for numerical data.

ANOVA

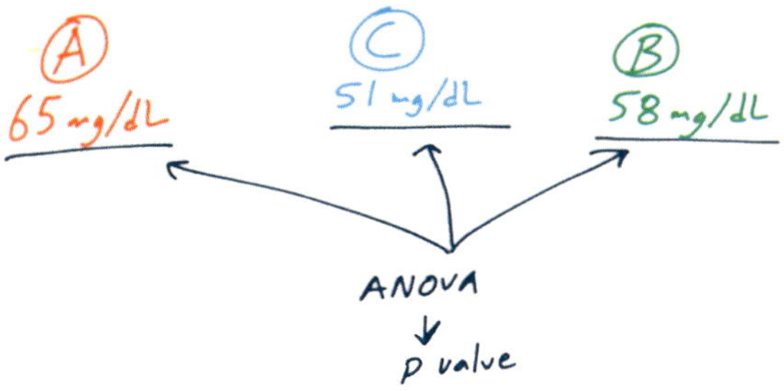

IV. Chi-square Test

A. Can find associations.

B. Used for categorical data (as opposed to numerical data).

1. Age, gender, race
2. Treated v not treated
3. High or Low

C. Percentages can be used for categorical data.

1. Example: 35% of heavy smokers. Being a "heavy smoker" is categorical.

Chi-Square

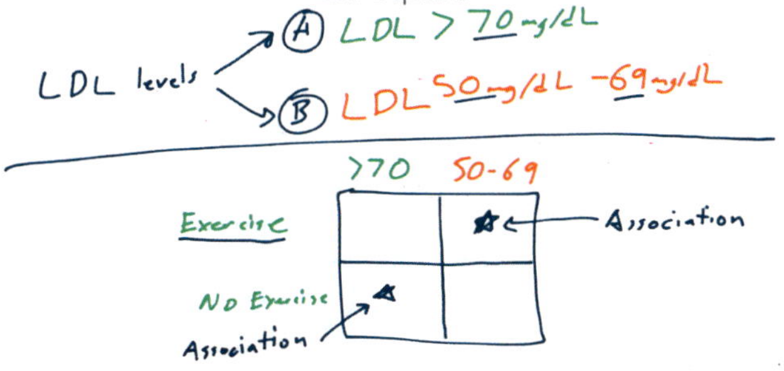

V. Correlation Coefficient (r)

A. Evaluates relationship (correlation) between two variables.

B. Ranges from -1 to +1.

C. Direction determined by (+) or (-).

D. Strength determined by numerical value (0 to 1).

E. Often demonstrated in scatter plots.

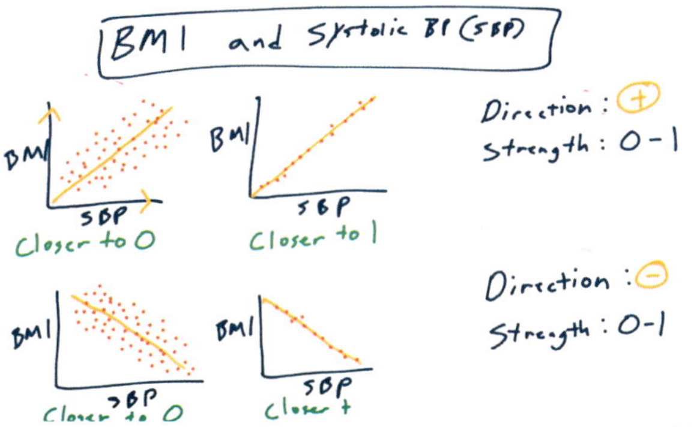

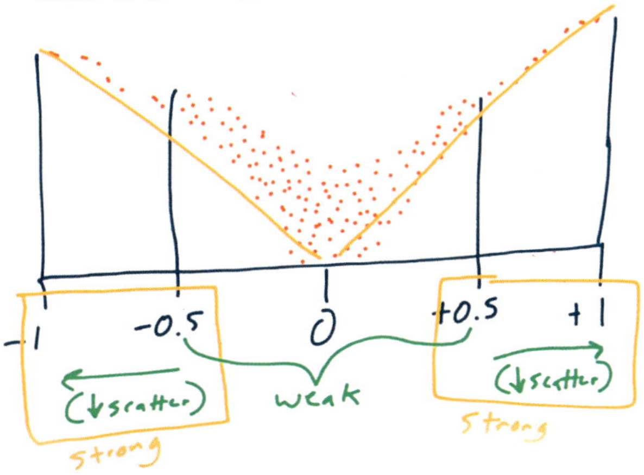

VI. Meta-Analysis

A. Meta-analysis analyzes the pooled data of many studies.

B. Collective data → higher sample size (n) → higher statistical power than studies individually.

C. Statistical power should make you think low β (power = 1 - β).

REVIEW QUESTIONS ?

1. The serum testosterone level of 150 males between the ages of 30 to 69 were measured. The males were broken into two groups based on their age. Ages of the first group ranged from 30 to 49 and ages of the second group ranged from 50 to 69. What test would best evaluate the averages of both groups?

- **Rule out Chi-square test because testosterone is not measured as a categorical variable.**
- **Rule out ANOVA since only 2 groups are evaluated.**
- **Two-sample t test is correct since it compares the means of 2 groups.**

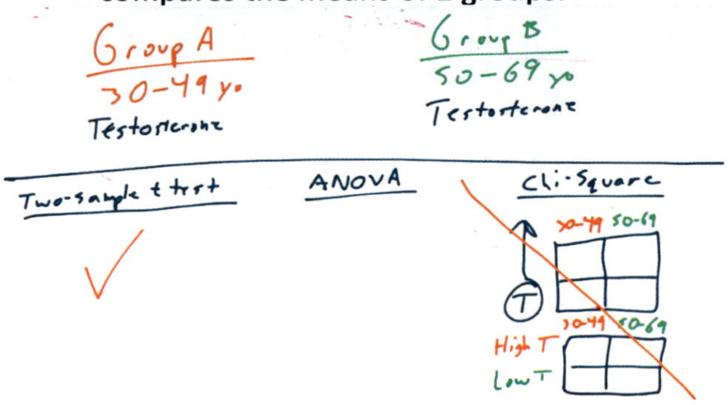

2. A study finds that higher use of cigarettes decreased the incidence of uterine cancer in postmenopausal women. Researchers also found that most cancer-free women did not smoke. What is the likely strength and direction of the correlation coefficient?

- **Direction is negative: increasing tobacco use with decreasing incidence of uterine cancer.**
- **Strength is weak: Most cancer-free patients did not smoke.**

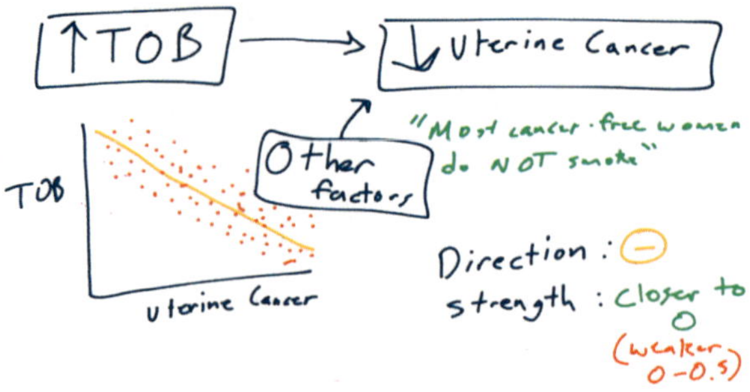

Section V - Bias and Confounders

I. Bias causes results to differ from reality.

II. Three broad categories:

A. Selection bias

B. Bias during experiment

C. Interpretation bias

III. Selection Bias

A. Bias that occurs because the pool of subjects does not represent general population.

1. Sampling Bias: Trial patients differ from clinical patients.

2. Berkson Bias: Only the sickest patients are enrolled.

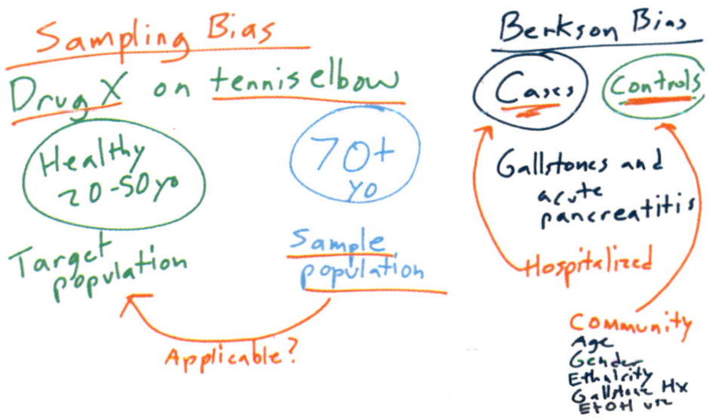

a) Non-response Bias: Enrollment different between groups.

b) Attrition Bias: Drop-out difference between groups.

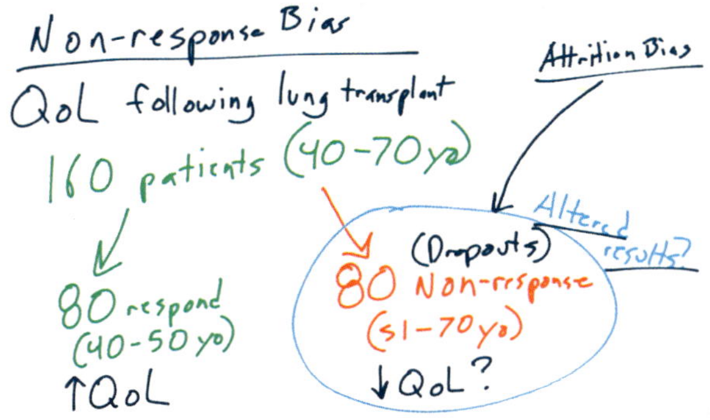

B. Bias During Experiment

1. Faulty data gathering during experiment → results differ from reality.

2. Can be thought of as arising from the researcher bias, measurement bias, or participant bias.

a) Researcher causes of bias during the experiment

(1) Observer-Expectancy Bias

(a) Investigator's prior knowledge influences data input.

(b) Reduce with blinding.

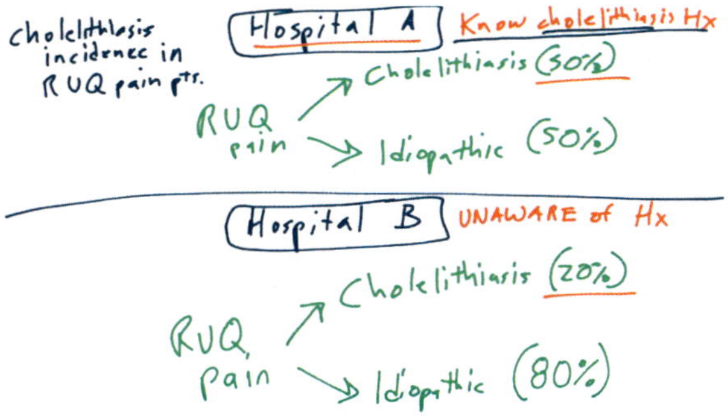

(2) Procedure Bias

(a) Participants are treated differently.

(b) Reduce with blinding.

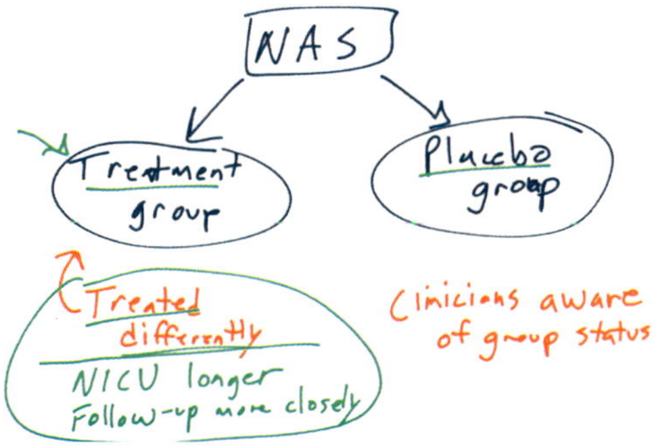

(3) Distinguish observer-expectancy and procedure bias based on data input versus treatment.

b) Measurement bias during the experiment

(1) Information gathered using equipment or mechanisms that are not standardized or otherwise faulty.

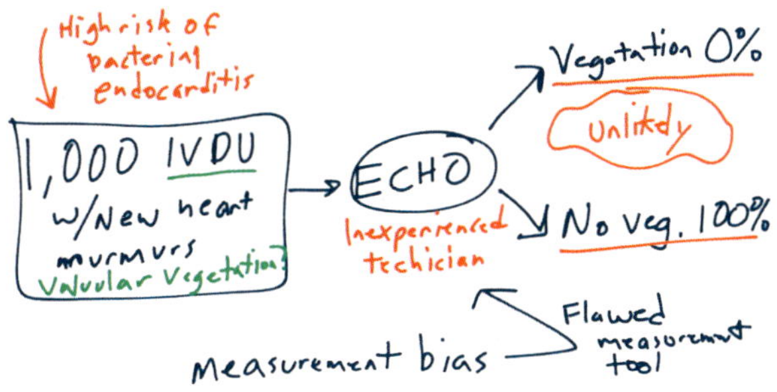

c) Participant causes of bias during the experiment

(1) Hawthorne Effect

(a) Subjects change their behavior upon learning they are being studied.

(b) Reduce with blinding.

(2) Recall Bias

(a) Patients with disease are more likely to recall past exposure.

(b) Reduce by decreasing time between the time at diagnosis and the time the study is performed.

(3) Reporting Bias

(a) Patients under or over report their experiences.

(b) Under-reporting could result from shame of disease and unwillingness to disclose all details.

(c) Over-reporting could result from emotional response to disease, thus overemphasizing symptoms.

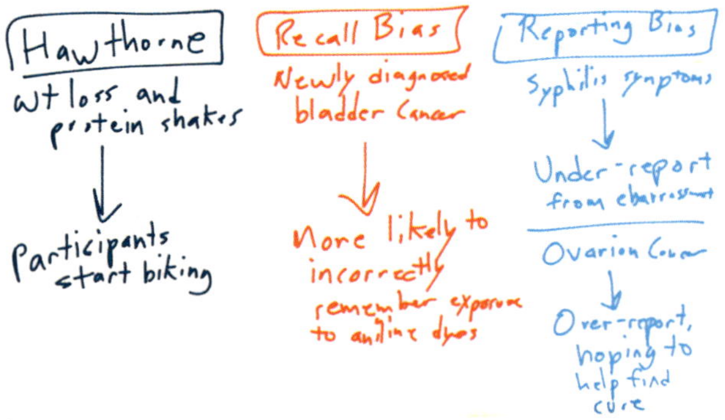

C. Interpretation Bias

1. Incorrect interpretation of study results or data analysis leading to bias.

2. Confounding Bias

a) An uncontrolled variable caused a difference to be seen when there is no difference.

b) Can be reduced with matching.

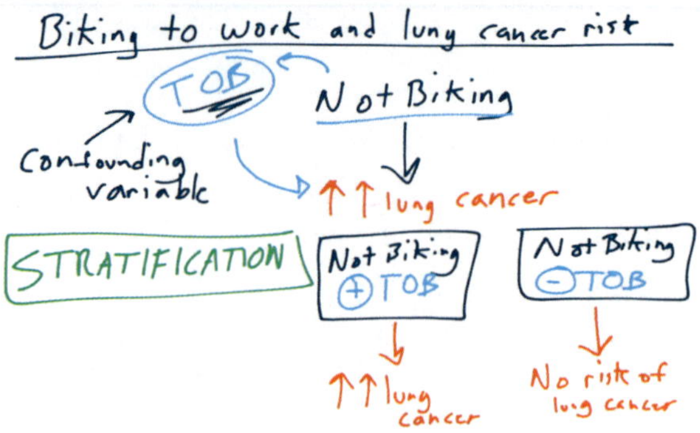

3. Effect Modification

a) Not considered a bias

b) Another variable increases or decreases the impact of a risk factor.

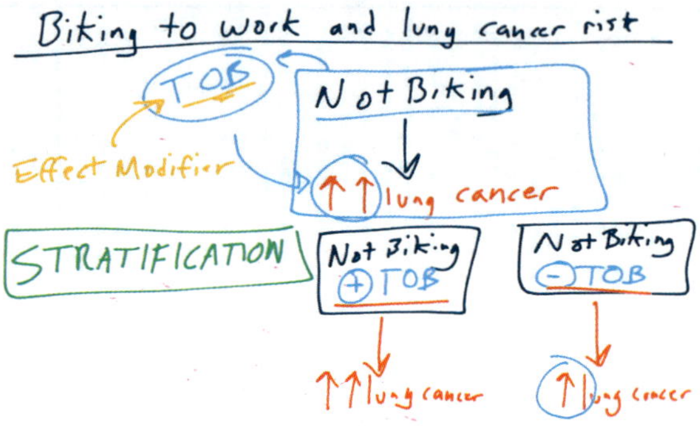

4. Confounding Bias and Effect Modification

a) Distinguished from confounding bias through stratifying.

b) If the relationship exists but it less drastic, it is effect modification.

c) If, after stratifying, there is no relationship, it is confounding bias.

5. Lead-time Bias

a) Mistakenly believing a screening test increases the survival of patients by catching a disease earlier.

b) A screening test that catches a disease earlier without altering its progression.

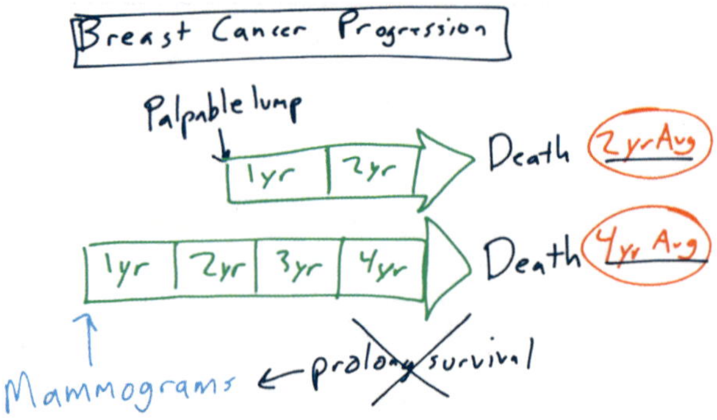

6. Length-time Bias

a) Slowly progressing diseases are caught more than rapidly progressing variations of the disease.

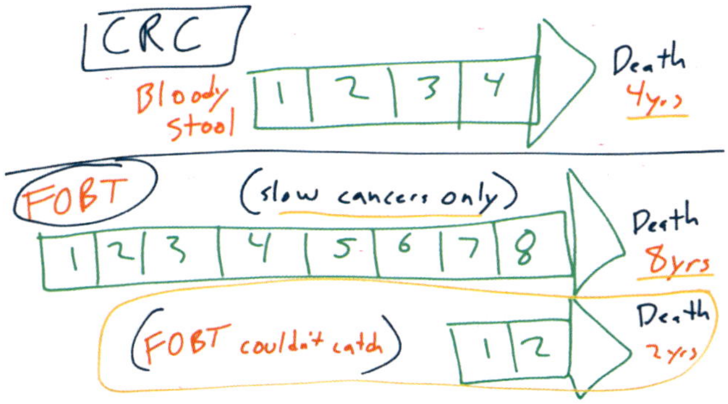

7. Lead-time Bias versus Length-time Bias

   a) Lead-time bias

      (1) Diagnose disease earlier

   b) Length-time bias

      (1) Diagnose more benign and fewer aggressive variations.

   c) Both mistakenly assume increased survival.

Section VI - Applying Studies to Patients: Sensitivity and Specificity

I. Introduction

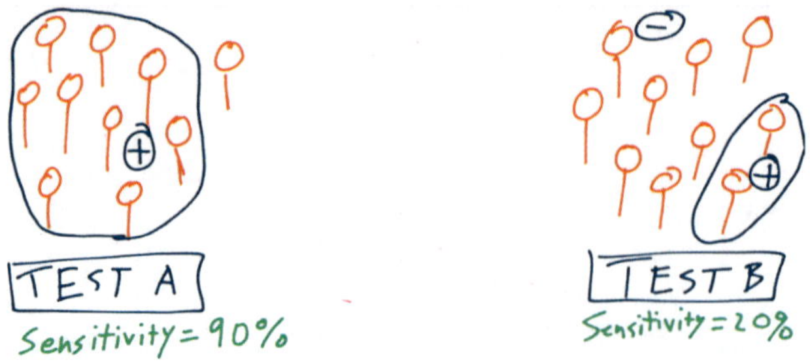

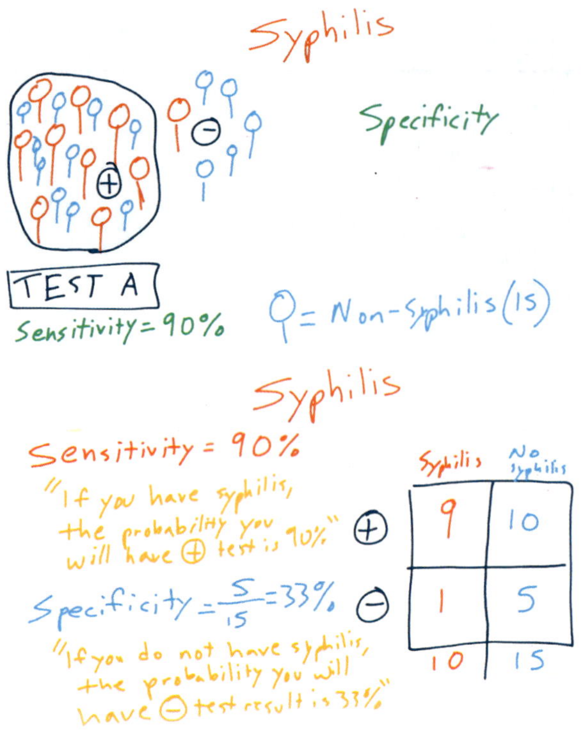

II. Sensitivity

A. If you have the disease, the probability that your test will be positive.

B. Technical math: true positives / (true positives + false negatives)

1. Use 2 x 2 table to plot out

C. Better way

1. Numerator = Diseased and Positive

2. Denominator = Diseased

III. Specificity

A. If you don't have the disease, the probability that your test will be negative

B. Technical math: true negatives / (true negatives + false positives)

1. Use 2 x 2 table to plot out

C. Better way

1. Numerator = Disease-free and Negative

2. Denominator = Disease-free

IV. Sensitivity and Specificity on a 2x2 Table

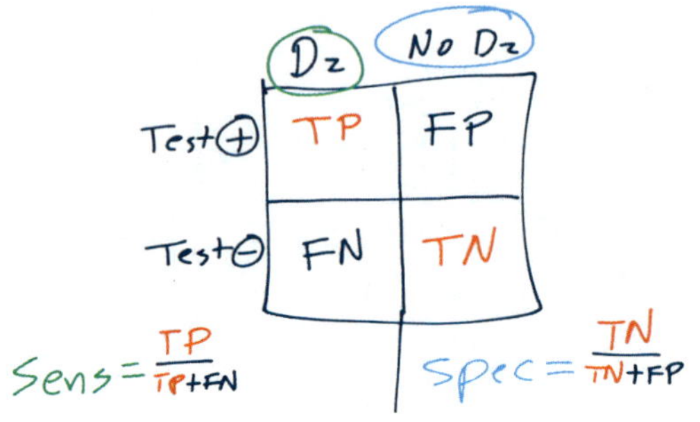

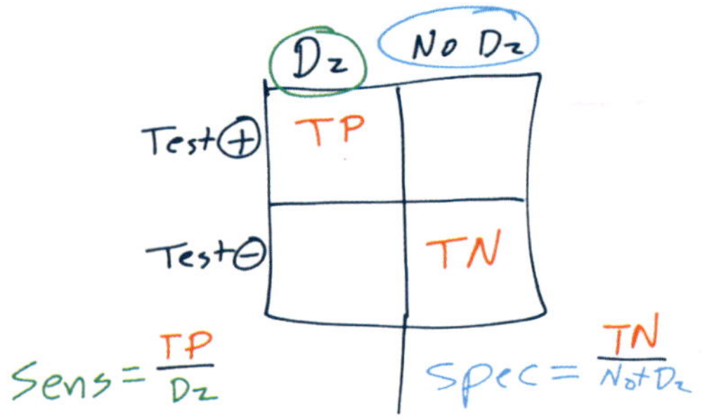

V. Sensitivity and Specificity on Graph

A. Ideal test: 100% sensitivity and 100% specificity (not realistic).

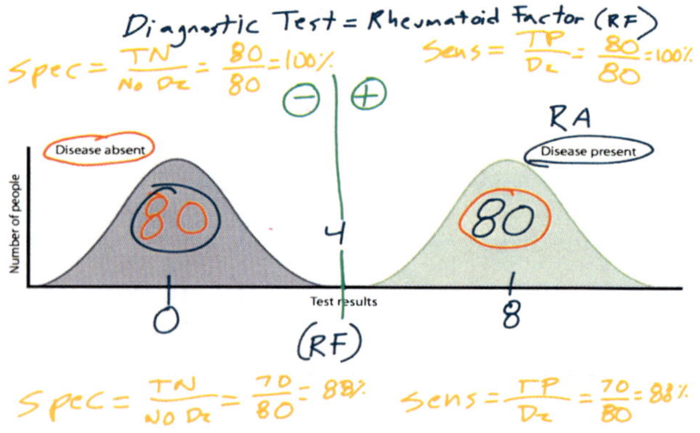

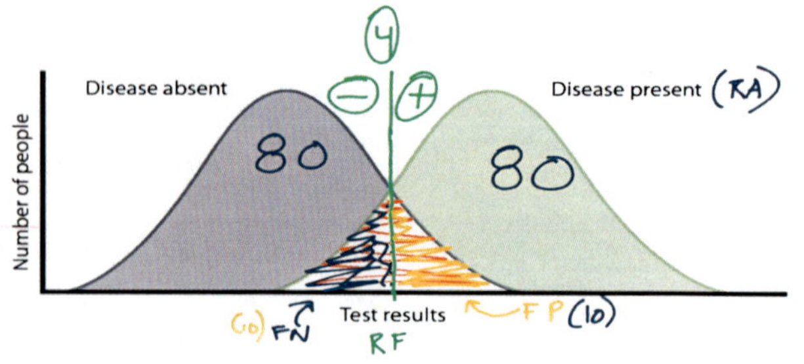

B. Moving diagnostic cut-off left

1. ↑ TP → ↑ sensitivity (sensitivity = TP / all diseased).
2. ↓ TN → ↓ specificity (specificity = TN / all disease-free).

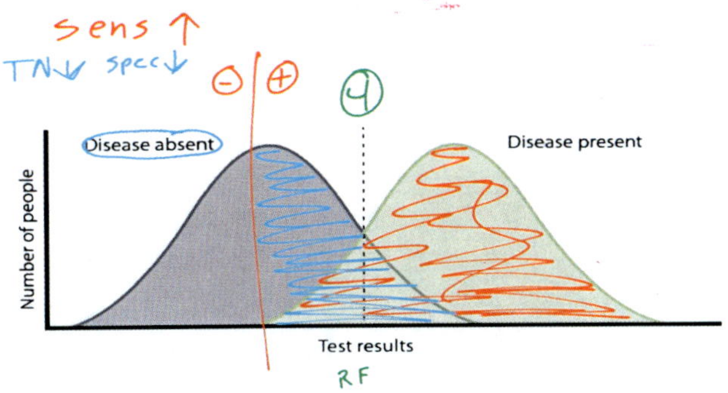

C. Moving diagnostic cut-off right

1. ↑ TN → ↑ specificity (specificity = TN / all disease-free).
2. ↓ TP → ↓ sensitivity (sensitivity = TP / all diseased).

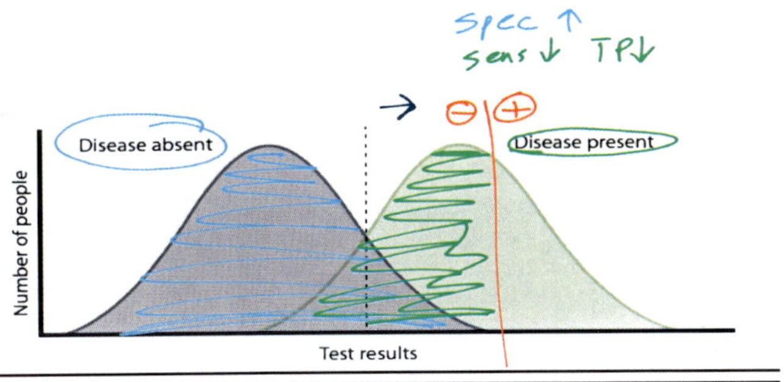

D. Specificity

1. 100% specific → + test → rule IN disease
2. "SpIN"

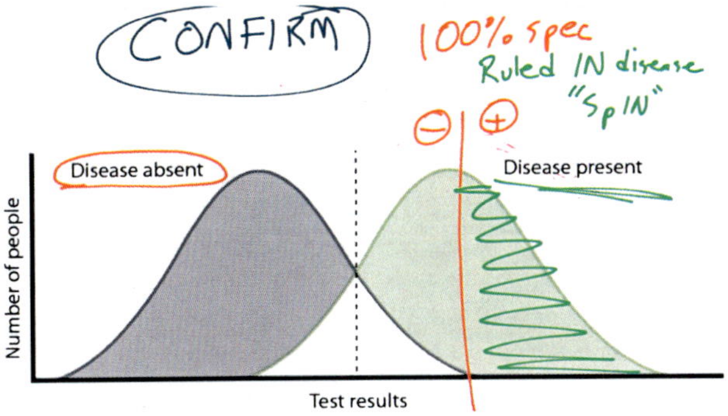

E. Sensitive

1. 100% sensitive → – test → rule OUT disease
2. "SnOUT"

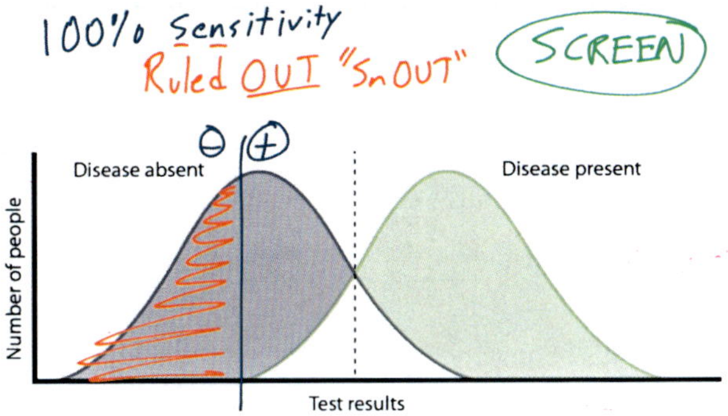

3. Typical pattern: Screen with sensitive test. Confirm with specific test.

F. Calculating False Negatives and False Positives

1. Specificity
   a) False positive (FP) percentage = 1 - Specificity
   b) Example: 75% specific → 25% are falsely positive (FP)
2. Sensitivity
   a) False negative (FN) percentage = 1 - Sensitivity
   b) Example: 82% sensitive → 18% are falsely negative (FN)

REVIEW QUESTIONS

1. A research group is trying to determine how valuable test X will be for diagnosing hepatocellular carcinoma (HCC). There are 800 patients in the study. Of those, 250 have confirmed HCC. Of the diseased patients, 100 test positive with text X. The remaining participants test negative. What is the sensitivity of test X?

   - **Sensitivity = TP / diseased patients → 100 / 250 → 0.4 (40%)**

800 pts
250 HCC (100 test ⊕) ↑ TP

Test X sensitivity $= \frac{TP}{Dz} = \frac{100}{250} = 0.4 (40\%)$

"Test X will only catch 40% of all HCC patients"

	HCC	No HCC
Test ⊕	100	
Test ⊖	150	
	250	

$Sens = \frac{100}{100+150}$

2. Using the above example, what is the specificity of text X?

   - **Specificity = TN / Non-diseased patients → 550 / 550 → 1.0 (100%)**

(all of them) 550

800 total − 250 HCC = 550 No Dz

Only 100 test ⊕ (all HCC)

Specificity of Test X $= \frac{TN}{No\ Dz} = \frac{550}{550} = 1 (100\%)$

	HCC	No Dz
Test ⊕		0
Test ⊖		550
		550

"If you don't have the disease, the probability you will test ⊖ is 100%

3. The sensitivity of diagnostic test Y is 40% while the specificity is 100%. Which cut-off value, indicated by the yellow bar, accurately depicts diagnostic test Y?

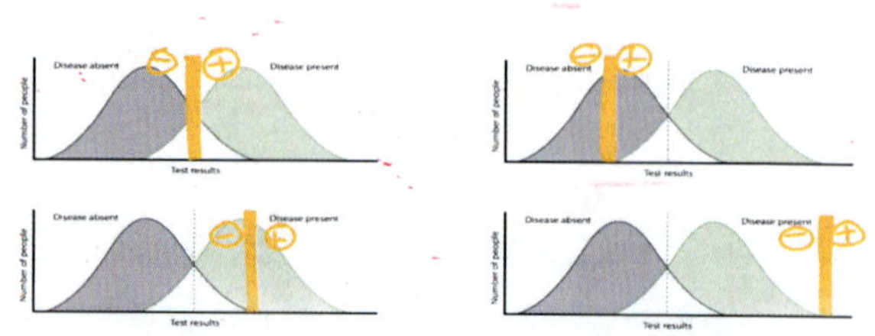

   - **100% specificity means all disease-free patients test negative → top two options can be ruled out.**
   - **40% sensitivity indicates that at least some diseased patients show up positive → the bottom right option can be ruled out.**

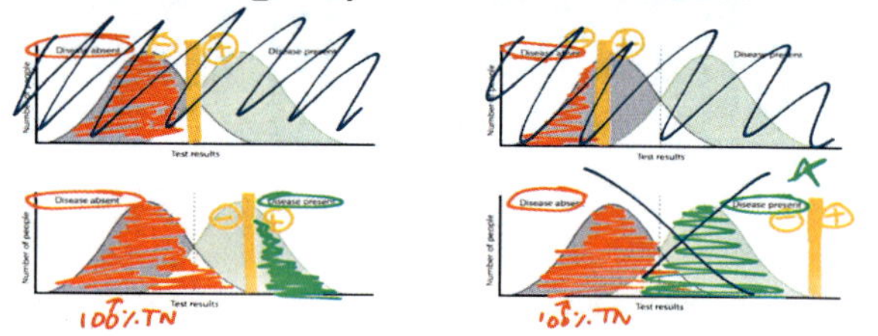

4. You suspect one of your patients has Disease K, a very rare disease. You want to be sure you don't miss it, so you order Test B. The results come back negative. Based on what you know about Test B, you now feel confident your patient is free of Disease K. Was the test highly sensitive or specific?

   - **If you feel confident your patient does not have the disease following a negative test, then you ruled out a disease → highly sensitive test**

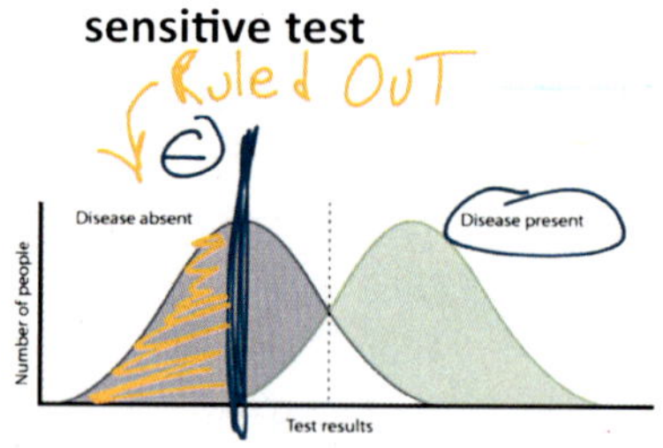

⊖ Test → Confident your patient is free of Disease K
Ruled OUT "SnOUT"

REVIEW QUESTIONS ?

5. Five hundred obese patients received a screening test for hyperlipidemia. The screening test is 60% specific and 90% sensitive. How many of these patients will be falsely positive?

- **False positive = 1 - specificity (0.6 in this case) → 0.4 (40%) of participants must test falsely positive (FP) → 0.4 x 500 patients → 200**

500 patients
Sens= 90%
Spec = 60%

FP= 1 − spec
1 − 0.6
0.4 (40%)
↑
40% are falsely ⊕

0.4 x 500 = 200

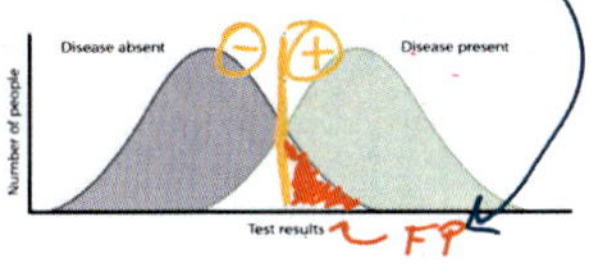

Section VII - PPV and NPV

I. Positive Predictive Value (PPV)

A. If you have a positive test, the probability that you will have the disease.

B. PPV increases with increased prevalence.

C. Technical way: True positive / (True positive + False positive)

D. Better way

1. Numerator = positive test result AND diseased

2. Denominator = positive test result

$PPV = \frac{TP}{TP+FP} = \frac{TP}{\oplus}$

"If you have ⊕ test, PPV tells you the probability of having the Disease"

	Dz	No Dz
Test ⊕	TP	FP
Test ⊖	FN	TN

II. Negative Predictive Value (NPV)

A. The probability that you will not have the disease if you test negative.

B. NPV increases with *decreased* prevalence.

C. Technical way: True negative / (True negative + False negative)

D. Better way

1. Numerator = negative test result AND not diseased

2. Denominator = negative test result

$NPV = \frac{TN}{TN+FN} = \frac{TN}{\ominus}$

"If you have ⊖ test, NPV tells you the probability you do not have the disease"

	Dz	No Dz
Test ⊕		
Test ⊖	FN	TN

III. Relating PPV and NPV to Prevalence

A. PPV increases as the prevalence increases

B. NPV increases as the prevalence decreases

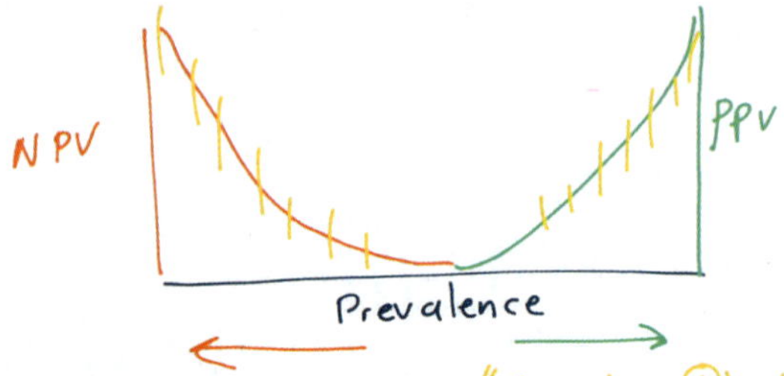

"If you test ⊖, NPV tells you the prob. you DO NOT have the disease"

"If you have ⊕ test, PPV tells you the prob. you will have the disease"

IV. Relating PPV and NPV to Sensitivity and Specificity

A. Specificity and PPV

1. Specificity α 1/FP α PPV

	Dz	No Dz
⊕		FP
⊖		

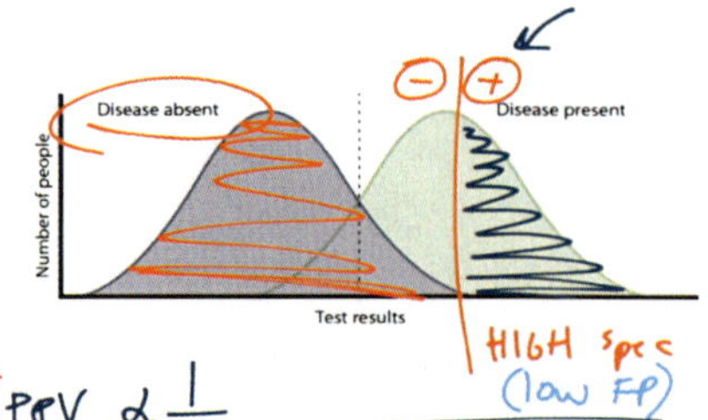

↑Spec α ↑PPV α 1/↓FP

HIGH Spec (low FP)

PPV = "If you test ⊕, PPV tells you prob. you have the disease"

B. Sensitivity and NPV

1. Sensitivity α 1/FN α NPV

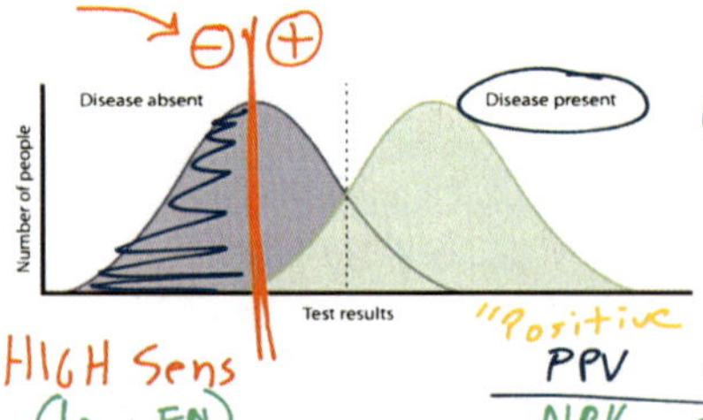

	Dz	No Dz
⊕		
⊖	FN	

HIGH Sens (low FN)

"Positive specs are falsely pos."

PPV — Spec — 1/FP

NPV — Sens — 1/FN

NPV = "If you get ⊖ test, NPV tells you probability of NOT having the disease"

C. Mnemonic: "Positive specs are falsely positive"

REVIEW QUESTIONS

1. There are 350 patients with suspected polymyositis who are tested by measuring serum anti-Jo-1 antibodies. There are 100 patients with a negative test, but 50 of them do not have polymyositis. The remaining 250 patients are positive, 150 of which do not have polymyositis. What is the positive predictive value of this test (PPV)?

   - **PPV = TP / Positive tests → 100 / 250 = 0.4 (40%)**

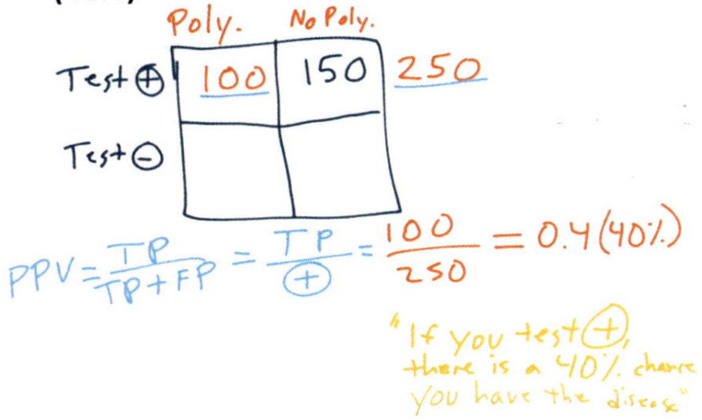

2. The negative predictive value of test A is 80%. One thousand patients test negative. What number of these patients are false negatives?

   - **NPV = TN / negative test results → 80% = (0.8 x 1,000) / 1,000**
   - **FN = 1,000 - 800 = 200 false negatives**

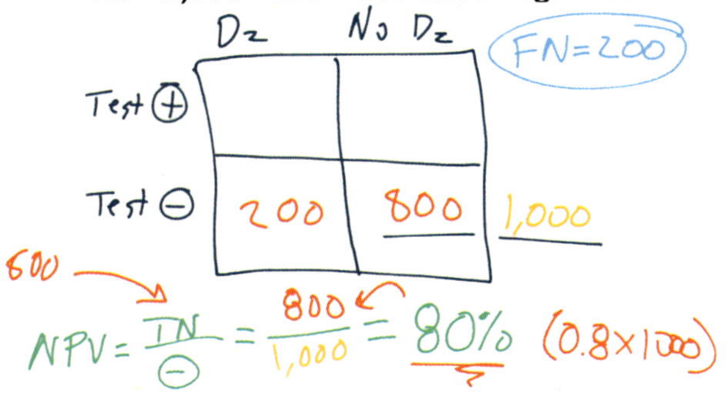

3. Two men undergo a test that screens for Malaria. Man A lives in the United States. Man B lives in southeast Asia. If both men have a negative test, which one is more likely to be disease free?

   - **The question is referring to NPV**
   - **Assume malaria is more prevalent in SE Asia → lower NPV**
   - **Lower prevalence in USA → higher NPV (a negative test more likely to indicate disease-free status)**

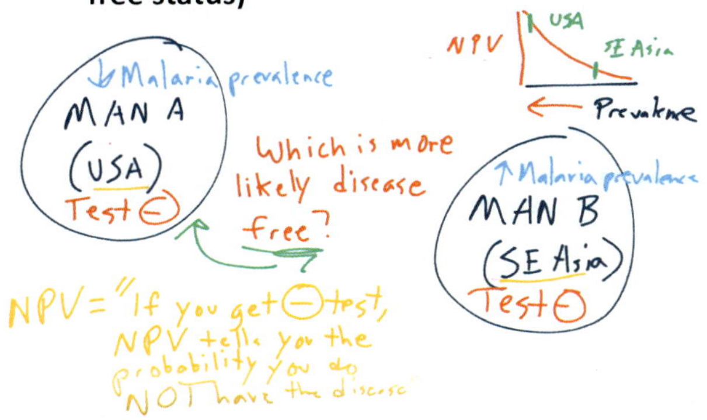

4. An ongoing research study is evaluating a diagnostic test. Early in the study (time A), a preliminary calculation finds the specificity to be 90%. The study continues and reexamination of the data two years later (time B) finds that the specificity has decreased. What happened to the PPV and the false positive rate from time A and time B?

   - **Specificity decreased from time A to time B**
   - **Recall mnemonic: "Positive specs are falsely positive"**
   - **If specificity decreased, PPV must have decreased and FP must have increased**

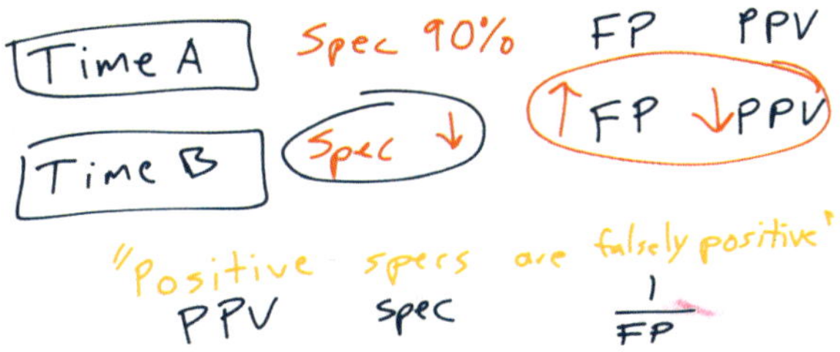

Section VIII - Likelihood Ratios, Incidence, and Prevalence

I. Incidence

A. New cases during time X / Population at risk

B. Note: patients diseased prior to time X are not at risk.

C. Found in cohort studies.

II. Prevalence

A. Total cases / Population

B. Found in cross-sectional studies (or ecological studies).

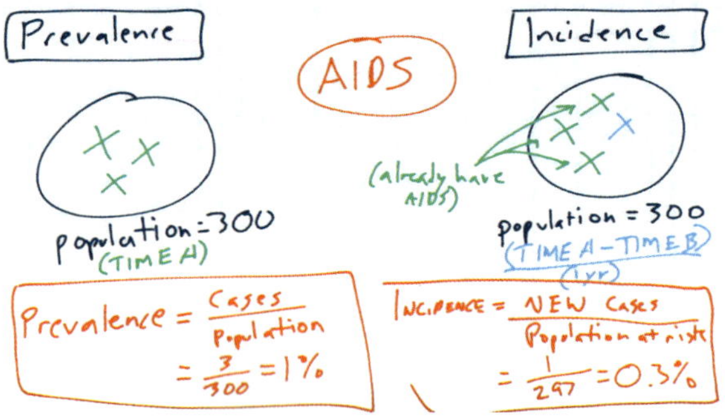

III. Relating Prevalence to Sensitivity, Specificity, LR, PPV and NPV

A. ↑ Prevalence → ↑ PPV

B. ↓ Prevalence → ↑ NPV

C. Prevalence does NOT impact sensitivity, specificity or likelihood ratios

IV. Likelihood Ratio (LR)

A. Positive LR (LR+) = How much probability of disease *shifts up* if test result is positive.

1. Ideal test: LR+ > 10

B. Negative LR (LR-) = How much probability of no disease *shifts down* if test result is negative.

1. Ideal test: LR- < 0.1 (i.e. less than 10% of current risk)

C. Must know pre-test probability.

D. All tests have a LR+ and a LR-

E. Calculate LR+ to evaluate the impact of a positive test.

F. Calculate LR- to evaluate the impact of a negative test.

G. If the likelihood ratios would not change treatment, don't order the test.

H. Likelihood Ratio and Sensitivity and Specificity

1. LR+ = Sensitivity / (1 - specificity)

2. LR- = (1 - sensitivity) / specificity

3. Not altered by prevalence.

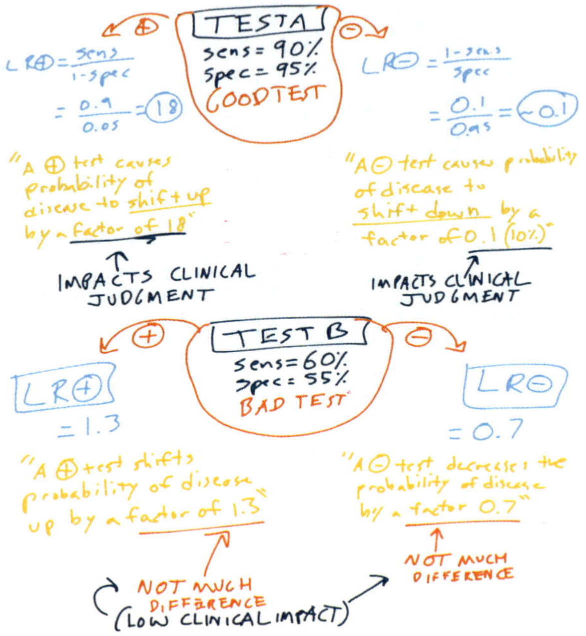

V. Likelihood Ratio vs. PPV and NPV

A. Likelihood ratios tell you *shift* in probability.

1. LR+ = If you get + test, your probability *shifts up by X.*

2. LR- = If you get - test, your probability *shifts down by X.*

B. Predictive values tell you *current* probability.

1. PPV = If you get + test, your probability of having disease *is Y.*

2. NPV = If you get - test, your probability of not having disease *is Y.*

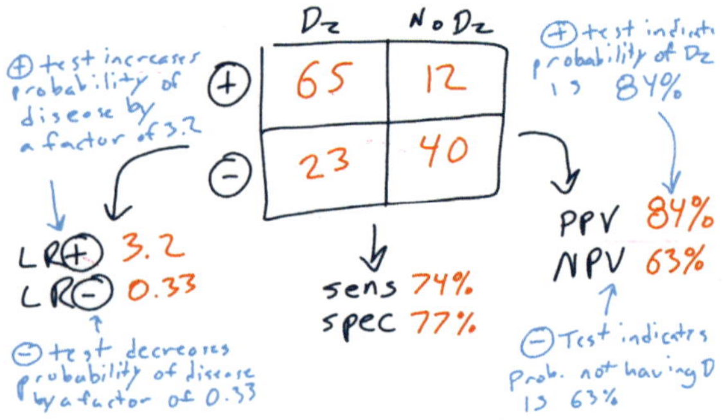

REVIEW QUESTIONS ?

1. A woman is told by her physician that she may have disease M. However, the physician warns that the test used to diagnose disease M does a poor job of catching all the diseased patients. Even with this knowledge, the woman would like to have the test performed and claims that the disease is now more common in her community. If the disease is more common in her community, what impact would this have on the probability of the test coming back positive if she has disease M?

   - **The question stem describes a test with low sensitivity**
   - **Prevalence does not alter sensitivity**

Disease M

"If you have the disease, the probability of a ⊕ test is low" (Low Sensitivity)

Test does a poor job catching all diseased pts

NOPE !!

Disease M ↑ prevalence

Prevalence → NPV, PPV

Prevalence does NOT impact Sensitivity, Specificity, LRs

2. An 82-year-old male with suspected acute myelogenous leukemia (AML) is about to undergo diagnostic test F. Prior to suggesting this test to the patient, the physician studies the literature and finds that a positive test increases the patient's odds of AML by a factor of 11.3. However, a negative test indicates the patient's chance of not having AML is 0.8. What information was given by the values of 11.3 and 0.8?

   - **11.3 describes the LR+**
   - **0.8 describes the NPV**

⊕ test ↑ odds of AML × 11.3 LR⊕

⊖ test indicates probability of NOT having AML is 0.8 (80%) NPV

Section IX - Measurements of Risk

I. Measurements of Risk Overview

A. Identifies risk of disease based on exposure.

B. Exposure may increase or reduce risk.

C. Require *p* value to reveal statistical significance.

D. Use 2 x 2 contingency table.

E. Information can be used to find many measurements.

1. Risk
2. Relative risk (RR)
3. Odds ratio (OR)
4. Attributable risk
5. Relative risk reduction (RRR)
6. Absolute risk reduction (ARR)
7. Number needed to treat (NNT)
8. Number needed to harm (NNH)

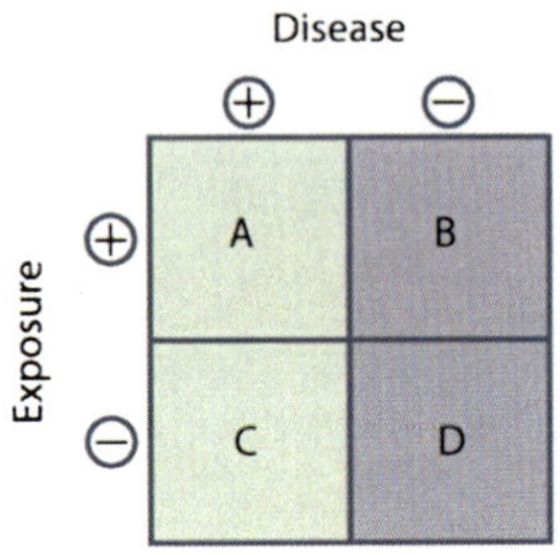

II. Risk Definition

A. Risk of disease in exposed

1. A / (A + B)
2. Risk = incidence

B. Risk of disease in unexposed

1. C / (C + D)
2. Risk = incidence

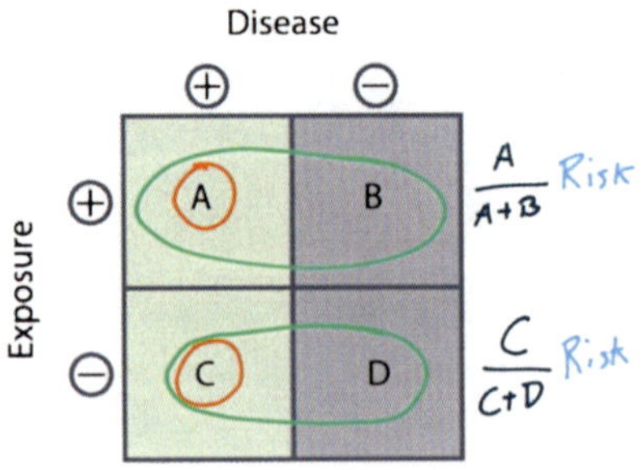

III. Relative Risk (RR)

A. Definition

1. If you have the exposure (or risk factor), the risk that you will develop the disease.
   a) I.e. your risk, relative to those who have not been exposed.
2. Used in cohort studies.

B. Calculation

1. RR = [a/(a+b)] / [c/(c+d)]
2. RR = Risk in exposed / Risk in unexposed.
3. RR = Incidence in exposed / Incidence in not exposed.

Sexually active young adults

RR of Chlamydia in those not using protection

Exposure = No protection: 200/1,000 = 0.2 (20%)

Unexposed = Use protection: 10/1,000 = 0.01 (1%)

RR = risk in exposed / risk in unexposed = 20% / 1% = 20

C. Associations

1. RR = 1 (null value) = no association
2. RR > 1 (positive association: exposure increases disease risk)
3. RR < 1 (negative association: exposure decreases disease risk)

RR > 1	RR < 1	RR = 1
No prot. / Protection: 20/1 = 20	No prot. / Protection: 1/20 = 0.05	No prot. / Protection: 20/20 = 1
"Not using protection increases chlamydia risk"	"Not using protection decreases risk of chlamydia" (ludicrous)	"Exposure does not alter risk of chlamydia"

IV. Odds Ratio (OR)

A. The odds that you were exposed if you have the disease.

B. Found in case-control studies.

C. OR = (a/c) / (b/d) = ad / bc

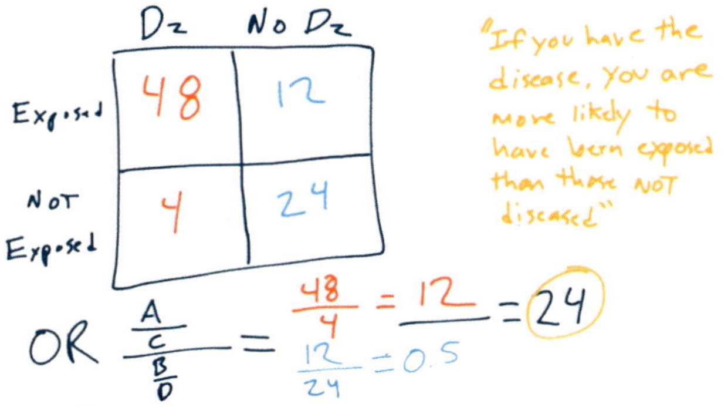

V. Odds Ratio (OR) versus Relative Risk (RR)

A. Relative Risk (superior)

1. Cohort studies
2. "You have the exposure? Here is your risk of getting disease."

B. Odds Ratio

1. Case-Control studies
2. "You have the disease? Here are the odds you were exposed."

C. OR ~ RR in rare diseases (prevalence < 10%)

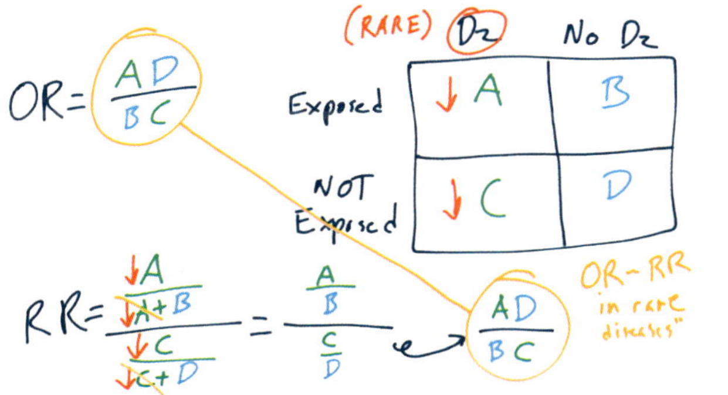

VI. Attributable Risk Percent (AR) and Number Needed to Harm (NNH)

A. Attributable Risk

1. The risk difference between exposed and unexposed individuals.
2. AR = risk in exposed - risk in unexposed
3. AR = a / (a+b) - c / (c+d)

B. Number Needed to Harm

1. The number of exposures needed for 1 disease outcome
2. NNH = 1 / AR

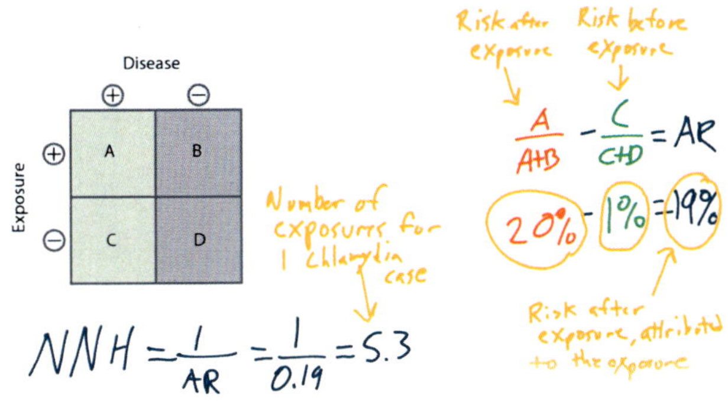

VII. Absolute Risk Reduction (ARR) and Number Needed to Treat (NNT)

A. Absolute Risk Reduction

1. The risk difference between treatment and control groups.
2. ARR = risk in treatment - risk in control
3. ARR = a / (a+b) - c / (c+d)

B. Number Needed to Treat

1. Number of treated people required to prevent 1 adverse outcome.
2. NNT = 1 / ARR

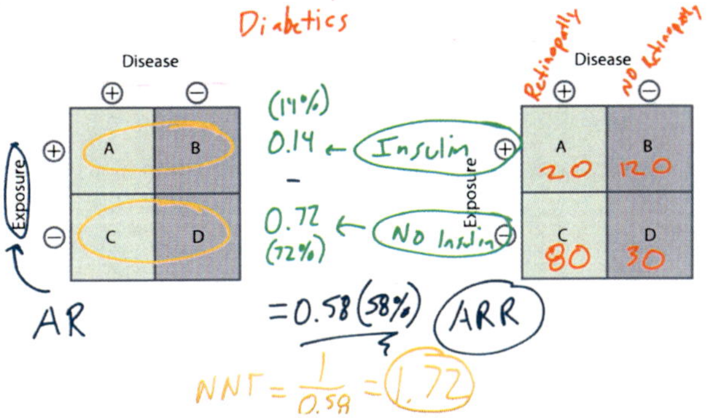

VIII. Relative Risk Reduction (RRR)

A. Relative difference between events in treatment versus control groups.

B. Found in cohort studies.

C. RRR = 1 - RR

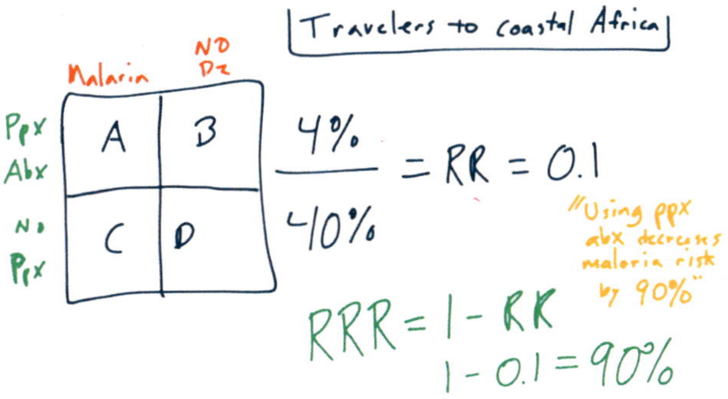

REVIEW QUESTIONS

1. An experiment finds that following exposure to substance B, the relative risk of developing disease X is 1.6 with a 95% CI (0.1 - 1.3). Describe the association between substance B and disease X.

   - **1.6 indicates a positive association, but the confidence interval includes 1, so there is no association**

RR = 1.6 (RR > 1) → Positive association

~~(Exposure to substance B increases risk of Disease X)~~

95% CI = 0.1 - 1.3

↳ INCLUDES 1 (Null value)

2. A study was performed after finding a group with disease Y. The exposure rate of toxin S was found in the group and their matched counterparts. Eighty-five diseased patients were exposed, while 25 diseased were not exposed. Out of the 105 individuals that were not diseased, 45 had been exposed. Calculate the association of disease Y to toxin S using the appropriate equation (RR or OR).

   - **First identify that the study type performed was a case-control study**
   - **Then find OR = 4.5**

Disease Y and Toxin S

OR

Toxin S: Diseased (cases)

Toxin S: Control group

(Case-Control)

	Dz Y	No Dz
Toxin S Exposure	85	45
No Exposure	25	60
		105

$OR = \frac{A/C}{B/D} = \frac{85/25}{45/60} = 4.5$

3. The incidence of bladder cancer in a large industrial factory over a 10 year period is 3%. The incidence of bladder cancer in the rest of the state is 0.5%. After some investigation, researchers determine that all of those factory workers were exposed to aniline dyes, a known risk factor for bladder cancer. How many exposures are required for 1 worker to develop bladder cancer.

   - **First find AR → 3% incidence - 0.5% incidence = 2.5% AR**
   - **NNH = 1 / AR = 1 / 0.025 = 40 exposed people**

Exposure = Aniline Dyes

Disease = Bladder Cancer

$NNH = \frac{1}{AR} = \frac{1}{0.025} = 40$

AR = Risk in exposed (incidence) 3% − Risk in unexposed (incidence) 0.5% = 2.5% (0.025)

Made in United States
North Haven, CT
05 November 2026

21765330R00018